PAGET'S DISEASE OF BONE RECIPES FOR BEGINNERS

Delicious Recipes, Foods, Meal Plans, And Expert Tips Designed To Alleviate Paget's Disease Discomfort And Promote Bone Healing

DR. JACE ZAYDEN

Table of Contents

DISCLAIMER

The information provided in the book is intended for general informational purposes only. The content of this book should not be considered a substitute for professional medical advice, diagnosis, or treatment.

Readers are advised to consult with a qualified healthcare professional for medical advice tailored to their individual circumstances.

The author has made every effort to ensure that the information in this book is accurate and up-to-date at the time of publication. However, medical knowledge is constantly evolving, and new research may emerge that could impact the information presented. The author disclaims any responsibility for any adverse effects or consequences resulting from the use of the information provided in this book.

References or mentions of individuals, products, websites, organizations, or other names within this book are for informational purposes only and do not constitute an endorsement. The author has no affiliations with, and makes no endorsements of, any third-party entities mentioned. Readers are encouraged to conduct their own research and exercise their judgment when considering any external resources or recommendations.

The author and the publisher shall have neither liability nor responsibility to any person or entity with respect to any loss, damage, or injury caused or alleged to be caused directly or indirectly by the information contained in this book. Any reliance on the information within this book is at the reader's own risk.

By reading this book, the reader acknowledges and agrees to the terms of this disclaimer. If the reader does not agree with these terms, they should not use the information provided in this book.

ABOUT THIS BOOK

"Paget's Disease of Bone Recipes" is an essential manual that explores the complex interplay between diet, way of life, and Paget's Disease of Bone management. An extensive introductory section commences this book, providing a foundational framework for comprehending the intricacies of this skeletal disorder. This book provides a comprehensive analysis of Paget's Disease, including diagnostic and medical management aspects. By doing so, it equips readers with vital information that enables them to effectively navigate the condition's complexities.

This book extensively addresses the significance of nutrition and dietary factors in Paget's Disease. The reader is instructed on the significance of calcium and vitamin D, which are essential nutrients for the preservation of bone health. The nutritional value of the content is enhanced through the incorporation of anti-inflammatory foods and bone-boosting recipes, which offer practical strategies for individuals who are afflicted with Paget's Disease.

This book provides a comprehensive approach by presenting effortless meal suggestions and culinary advice that are specifically designed for individuals diagnosed with Paget's Disease. Hydration is regarded as an essential component in the management of the condition. Furthermore, this book offers a methodical manual for devising meals to maximize bone health.

This book delves into the significance of consulting with healthcare professionals, acknowledging the criticality of collaboration in the healthcare industry. It promotes the adoption of a multidisciplinary strategy in the management of Paget's Disease, encouraging patients and healthcare providers to collaborate in this endeavor.

Furthermore, "Paget's Disease of Bone Recipes" encompasses lifestyle adjustments specifically designed for individuals afflicted with Paget's Disease, in addition to dietary recommendations. The incorporation of a segment devoted to frequently inquired questions (FAQs) serves to augment the reader's comprehension and functions as a valuable asset for individuals in search of elucidation regarding diverse facets of the condition. Fundamentally, this book functions as an all-encompassing and pragmatic manual, providing individuals afflicted with Paget's Disease and their attendants with the information and resources essential for effectively navigating the intricacies of condition management.

CHAPTER ONE

EXPLORING PAGET'S DISEASE OF THE BONE AND RECIPES FOR OPTIMAL HEALTH: NOURISHING WELL-BEING

Introduction

A chronic condition, Paget's Disease of Bone is distinguished by the atypical remodeling of bone tissue. The disease, which bears the name Sir James Paget, perturbs the typical equilibrium between bone formation and degradation, resulting in bones that are weakened and deformed. While the precise etiology is still unknown, it is hypothesized that genetic predispositions and environmental influences play a role in its progression.

Comprehension Of Paget's Disease Of The Bone:

Paget's Disease is more prevalent in the elderly demographic, where it primarily impacts the elderly. The condition has the potential to affect multiple bones, frequently affecting the pelvis, spine, cranium, and long bones. Although a considerable proportion of those afflicted with Paget's Disease may remain asymptomatic, certain individuals may manifest symptoms including bone pain, deformities, fractures, and in severe cases, hearing loss, if the cranium is affected.

Paget's Disease is characterized by aberrant bone remodeling, which entails an expedited decomposition of bone tissue and an exaggerated endeavor at restoration, culminating in bones that are structurally compromised. A variety of complications may result from this atypical skeletal configuration, such as arthritis, pain, and an elevated susceptibility to fractures.

Medical Diagnosis And Treatment:
To diagnose Paget's Disease, imaging studies, laboratory tests, and clinical evaluation are utilized in tandem. Blood tests, bone imaging, and X-rays can assist in confirming the diagnosis and determining the extent of bone involvement.

The objective of medical management, following a diagnosis, is to mitigate symptoms, avert complications, and enhance the overall health of the bones.

Bisphosphonates, which inhibit bone resorption, are frequently prescribed for the treatment of Paget's Disease. By inhibiting the aberrant bone remodeling process, these medications alleviate pain and prevent the development of additional deformities. Occasionally, surgical intervention may be required to treat complications such as joint injury or fractures.

Consistent monitoring, including blood and imaging analyses, is essential for determining the efficacy of treatment and making necessary adjustments to maintenance.

Although medical interventions remain essential, a comprehensive approach to Paget's Disease encompasses lifestyle elements, such as dietary and nutritional considerations.

Dietary And Nutritional Considerations:

Ensuring optimal nutrition is of utmost importance for individuals diagnosed with Paget's Disease, as it can serve to complement medical interventions and promote overall health. For optimal bone health, adequate calcium and vitamin D intake is essential. A lack of these essential nutrients can worsen the consequences of Paget's Disease, which affects bone density and mineralization.

To ensure sufficient calcium consumption, it is advisable to include a diverse range of dairy products, verdant green vegetables, fortified foods, and supplements in one's diet. Vitamin D supplementation, sun exposure, and consumption of oily fish are all crucial for the maintenance of adequate vitamin D levels. Calcium and vitamin D are both beneficial in promoting bone health and reducing the likelihood of fractures.

Paget's disease patients must consume a well-balanced diet that is abundant in vital nutrients.

The protein found in plant-based foods, fish, meat, and dairy products promotes healthy muscles and bones. Sustaining a healthy body weight is equally crucial, given that excessive weight can exacerbate symptoms by imposing further strain on the bones.

In addition to promoting bone health via nutrition, Paget's Disease patients must also effectively manage inflammation. Incorporating anti-inflammatory foods into one's diet, such as fatty salmon, almonds, fruits, and vegetables, can aid in the reduction of inflammation and promote general health.

Health-Optimal Recipes:

Meal preparation that places a premium on bone health and general well-being is a crucial component of Paget's Disease management. The following recipes have been meticulously crafted to meet the distinct nutritional requirements of individuals afflicted with Paget's Disease:

1. Spinach And Salmon Salad:

• Salmon fillets that have been grilled and are abundant in omega-3 fatty acids support inflammation.

• Fresh spinach to increase calcium intake.

• Finished with a lemon vinaigrette to impart vitamin C and enhance flavor.

2. Stir-Fried Quinoa And Vegetables:

Quinoa serves as a source of protein and vital amino acids that support bone health.

• Carrots, bell peppers, and broccoli are colorful vegetables that provide an assortment of vitamins and minerals.

• Garlic and ginger, which are recognized for their pro-inflammatory attributes, are stir-fried.

3. YOGURT Parfait In Greece:

• Greek yogurt, which is rich in calcium and protein.

• Fresh berries are incorporated for their antioxidant and vitamin content.

• Nuts were incorporated for a wholesome lipid boost.

In addition to satisfying the nutritional requirements of those with Paget's Disease, these recipes prioritize flavor and texture to enhance the dining experience. By integrating these recipes into a well-balanced diet in conjunction with medical management, individuals afflicted with Paget's Disease may experience an improvement in their overall quality of life and bone health.

An Analysis And Treatment Strategy

Paget's disease of bone is a persistent condition characterized by impaired bone remodeling, which ultimately results in the deformation and deterioration of bones. Paget's disease, so named after the physician who first described it in 1877, Sir James Paget, predominantly impacts the elderly population.

It is postulated that genetic factors and viral infections play a role in its development, although the precise etiology is still unknown.

Paget's disease is characterized by an excessively active bone remodeling process. Typically, bone tissue undergoes continuous degeneration and reconstruction. Paget's disease, on the other hand, disrupts this process, resulting in the development of atypical and enlarged skeletal structures. Areas that are frequently impacted consist of the pelvis, vertebrae, cranium, and long bones.

Although a considerable number of people with Paget's disease remain asymptomatic, others may encounter bone pain, rigidity in the joints, fractures, and other complications. Prompt identification is essential for efficient management. Frequently, blood tests, imaging studies such as X-rays, and, in certain instances, a bone biopsy are required for diagnosis.

Paget's disease is managed through a combination of pharmacotherapy and lifestyle adjustments. It is customary for physicians to prescribe bisphosphonates, including alendronate and risedronate, to reduce the rate of excessive bone resorption. In addition, physical therapy and pain management may be suggested to alleviate symptoms.

Ensuring a wholesome lifestyle is imperative for those who have been diagnosed with Paget's disease. Sufficient consumption of calcium and vitamin D is essential for maintaining optimal bone health. Weight-bearing activities, in particular, can aid in the maintenance of bone density and the prevention of fractures.

In conclusion, Paget's disease of the bone necessitates a holistic strategy encompassing both medical intervention and adjustments to one's lifestyle. Consistent monitoring and compliance with prescribed treatments are critical for the successful management of this condition and the preservation of an ideal standard of living.

The Value Of Vitamin D And Calcium In The Formation Of Strong Bones

Vitamin D and calcium are indispensable nutrients that are critical for the development and maintenance of healthy, robust bones. These two nutrients collaborate to facilitate calcium absorption and bone mineralization, among other physiological processes.

Calcium is a mineral that comprises a substantial proportion of the composition of bone. In addition to being critical for maintaining bone density and strength, it influences muscle activity, blood coagulation, and nerve communication. Insufficient calcium in the diet causes the body to withdraw calcium from the bones, which gradually weakens the structure of the bones.

Vitamin D, which is frequently called the "sunshine vitamin," is crucial for calcium absorption in the intestines. In addition, it aids in the regulation of blood calcium levels and promotes bone mineralization. Although sunlight stimulates the body's vitamin D production, supplementation and dietary intake are frequently required to meet recommended levels, particularly in regions with limited sunlight.

Particularly evident are the significance of calcium and vitamin D in conditions such as osteoporosis and Paget's disease of the bone. Because of a reduction in bone density, bones become more frail and susceptible to fractures in osteoporosis. In conjunction with weight-bearing exercises, adequate calcium and vitamin D consumption can aid in the prevention and management of osteoporosis.

As previously mentioned, Paget's disease is characterized by atypical bone remodeling; therefore, maintaining adequate levels of calcium and vitamin D is essential for promoting bone health and alleviating the disease's symptoms.

It is imperative to incorporate calcium-rich foods into one's diet, including dairy products, fortified foods, and verdant greens. Furthermore, the maintenance of optimal vitamin D levels is aided by dietary sources such as fortified foods, fatty fish, and exposure to sunlight.

In summary, a balanced dietary regimen comprising sufficient quantities of calcium and vitamin D, in conjunction with exposure to sunlight and, if required, dietary supplements, is essential for sustaining robust and healthy bones in old age.

CHAPTER TWO

Anti-Inflammatory Foods: Bone And Body Nourishment

While inflammation is an inherent physiological reaction of the body to damage and infection, persistent inflammation can give rise to a multitude of health complications, such as ailments affecting the bones. By including anti-inflammatory foods in one's diet, one can adopt a proactive stance toward promoting bone health and overall well-being.

Conditions that impact the joints and bones, such as rheumatoid arthritis, are associated with chronic inflammation. Additionally, the symptoms of Paget's disease and osteoporosis may be exacerbated by inflammation. A diet abundant in anti-inflammatory nutrients promotes a healthier immune system and aids in the reduction of inflammation.

Salmon and mackerel, which are both oily fish and are abundant in omega-3 fatty acids, are essential anti-inflammatory nutrients. It has been demonstrated that these fatty acids possess anti-inflammatory properties and potentially promote bone health. Additional sources of omega-3 fatty acids are hazelnuts, flaxseeds, and chia seeds.

Additionally, vibrant fruits and vegetables are excellent options. Antioxidants, which are found in cruciferous vegetables, berries, cherries, and verdant greens, aid in the fight against oxidative stress and inflammation.

Curcumin, the active ingredient in turmeric, imparts potent anti-inflammatory properties and can be integrated into a wide range of culinary preparations.

In addition to providing fiber and vital nutrients, whole cereals, nuts, and seeds are ingredients that support an anti-inflammatory diet. Olive oil may possess anti-inflammatory properties and is a healthful alternative to other cooking oils due to its monounsaturated fat content.

The inclusion of anti-inflammatory items in one's daily diet not only promotes the health of the bones but also enhances overall wellness. As they can contribute to inflammation, it is crucial to limit the intake of processed foods, refined carbohydrates, and saturated fats in excessive quantities.

In brief, the consumption of an anti-inflammatory diet that emphasizes whole, nutrient-dense foods aids in the mitigation of inflammation and promotes bone health. When combined with other lifestyle factors, this dietary approach can have a substantial impact on the prevention and management of skeletal system conditions.

Delightful And Nutrient-Dense Bone-Boosting Recipes

Bone health maintenance requires more than the use of supplements; it also requires the adoption of a nutritious and well-balanced diet. Including essential nutrients such as calcium, vitamin D, and anti-inflammatory components, bone-boosting recipes can be both delectable and nutritious.

1. Quinoa and Salmon Salad:

• Components:

• Fillets of grilled salmon

Quinoa, cooked

Both spinach and kale

Their-ripe tomatoes

• Sliced avocados

• Lemon and olive oil vinaigrette

This recipe integrates the nutritional advantages of salmon's omega-3 fatty acids for bone health with quinoa and verdant greens for protein and calcium. Olive oil and lemon vinaigrette contribute to the dish's anti-inflammatory properties and impart a surge of flavor.

2. Stir-Fried Vegetables with Tofu:

• Components:

Tofu cubes shall.

• Vivid bell peppers

For the broccoli florets

Carrots, cut into thin slices

Ginger and garlic

Soy sauce (2)

Tofu serves as a plant-derived calcium source, whereas the vibrant vegetables contribute an assortment of vitamins and antioxidants. Ginger and garlic contribute flavor and possibly anti-inflammatory properties.

3. YOGURT Parfait In Greece:

• Components:

Greek yogurt •

• Strawberries and blackberries combined

Granola, a

Drizzling honey

In addition to calcium and protein, the berries in Greek yogurt provide antioxidants. While providing a crispy component, the granola can also be enhanced with supplementary nutrients. A thin layer of honey imparts an inherent flavor.

4. Bowl of Turmeric Chicken and Quinoa:

• Components:

• Grilled chicken breast that has been turmeric-seasoned

Quinoa, a

• Roasted potato puree

Sautéed vegetables

• Tahini condiment

In contrast to the anti-inflammatory properties of turmeric-seasoned chicken, quinoa, and vegetables offer an assortment of vital nutrients.

The tahini dressing contributes healthful lipids and a creamy consistency.

5. Stuffed Spinach and Feta Mushrooms:

• Components:

• Extensive mushroom caps

Stir-fried spinach

Feta cheese, a

• Herbs and garlic

Olive oil •

Vitamin D is naturally present in mushrooms when they are exposed to sunlight. This dish, which is stuffed with sautéed spinach and feta, integrates savory elements with nourishing nutrients that support bone health.

By integrating these recipes for bone health into a balanced diet, individuals can enjoy a delectable and beneficial experience while also reducing their susceptibility to bone-related ailments. Together with other elements of a healthy lifestyle, such as consistent physical activity and exposure to sunlight, these recipes support a holistic approach to bone health.

An Analysis And Treatment Strategy

A chronic bone disorder, Paget's Disease of Bone is distinguished by atypical bone remodeling, which results in bones that are deformed and weakened. This malady, which was initially described by Sir James Paget in the 19th century, predominantly impacts the elderly population. The primary characteristic of Paget's Disease is the abnormally high rate of bone tissue degeneration and regrowth, which results in abnormally large and brittle bones.

Paget's Disease is characterized by a variety of symptoms, such as joint rigidity, deformities, and bone discomfort. It is postulated that Paget's Disease is influenced to some extent by both genetic and environmental factors, although the precise etiology of the condition remains unknown. Fortunately, several approaches exist for ameliorating the condition and enhancing the affected individuals' quality of life.

A vital component of Paget's Disease management is the maintenance of a healthy lifestyle, which includes a well-balanced diet that promotes bone health. Sufficient consumption of calcium and vitamin D is imperative, given their significant contributions to the strength and density of bones. Under the supervision of a medical professional, regular exercise can also aid in bone health maintenance and reduce the risk of fractures.

Medications may also be prescribed to soothe symptoms and modulate bone turnover, in addition to nutritional considerations.

The purpose of these medications is to restore a healthy equilibrium between the excessive formation and disintegration of bone that is characteristic of Paget's Disease.

Consistent monitoring and communication with healthcare providers are imperative for Paget's

Disease patients. This practice guarantees that any alterations in symptoms or general well-being can be promptly attended to, resulting in enhanced disease management and a higher standard of living.

CHAPTER THREE

Simple- Meals For Patients With Paget's Disease

A person with Paget's Disease of the Bone may experience difficulty comfortably chewing and swallowing. This may result in a difficult mealtime experience. However, with some forethought and ingenuity, it is possible to prepare nutritious and delectable meals that are simple to prepare.

A highly beneficial dietary choice for individuals afflicted with Paget's Disease is the integration of delicate and tender foods. Soups, stews, and casseroles are frequently more manageable to digest than solid foods and contain an assortment of nutrients.

Choosing fruits and vegetables that have been properly prepared and are thus amenable to mashing or pureeing is an additional method of guaranteeing a more tender consistency.

Protein is an essential dietary component, and individuals diagnosed with Paget's Disease must prioritize the consumption of milder protein sources. Tender meats, fish, eggs, and dairy products are all examples. The integration of protein-rich foods into one's diet is beneficial for overall health and muscle strength.

Individuals with chewing difficulties may benefit from texture-modified foods, including minced or coarsely diced items. These alterations facilitate the consumption of an extensive range of foods while maintaining adequate nutritional value. By utilizing culinary implements such as food processors and blenders, one can attain the intended consistency, thereby enhancing the dining experience.

In addition to altering the consistency of food, it is critical to consider flavors and seasonings. By imbuing milder foods with the flavors of herbs, seasonings, and flavorful sauces, individuals with Paget's Disease can be motivated to consume a more balanced diet.

It is imperative to consult with a registered dietitian or healthcare professional before meal planning for patients diagnosed with Paget's Disease. They are capable of offering customized guidance to an individual's unique dietary preferences and nutritional needs, thereby guaranteeing the fulfillment of nutritional obligations and resolving any difficulties associated with ingesting and digesting.

Cooking Advice For Patients With Paget's Disease

When preparing meals for people with Paget's Disease, substantial thought must be given to both their nutritional requirements and any physical obstacles they may encounter. The following cookery suggestions are intended to enhance the palatability and enjoyment of meals for individuals afflicted with Paget's Disease.

1. Select Tender Meat segments: When selecting meat, choose tender segments that necessitate minimal swallowing. By employing cooking techniques such as braising, gradual simmering,

or stewing, meat can be rendered more tender and chewily pleasant.

2. One should incorporate broths and stews that are abundant in nutrients, as they not only offer solace but also supply vital nutrients. To facilitate consumption, opt for alternatives that consist of well-cooked proteins and tender vegetables.

3. Make use of food processors and blenders: Individuals afflicted with Paget's Disease may find these household appliances indispensable. By employing them to puree or precisely mince ingredients, one can achieve more manageable textures.

4. Incorporate soft cereals and legumes, such as quinoa, or thoroughly cooked legumes, into your meal preparations. These alternatives contribute to dietary diversity while supplying vital nutrients.

5. Because cooked fruits and vegetables are typically milder than their raw counterparts, choose them. By softening them with steam,

simmering, or baking, they become more manageable to mastic.

6. The utilization of herbs and spices to augment flavor is an essential component in the creation of palatable meals. Spices, herbs, and flavorful condiments may be utilized to improve the flavor of milder foods.

7. Small, frequent meals should be prioritized over large meals. Strive to incorporate smaller, more frequent meals into your daily routine. This strategy can facilitate energy management and reduce the difficulty of consuming.

8. Maintaining proper hydration is critical for maintaining overall health, which includes the health of bones. It is imperative to provide Paget's Disease patients with convenient access to hydrating beverages, including water.

9. Engage the Services of a Dietitian or Nutritionist: Consult with a registered dietitian or nutritionist, both of whom are healthcare professionals, to develop an individualized meal

plan that addresses any specific challenges and fulfills the individual's nutritional requirements.

By integrating these culinary recommendations, people afflicted with Paget's Disease can partake in a varied and nourishing dietary regimen while mitigating the difficulties related to mastication and aspiration.

Suggestions And Critical Considerations

It is especially vital for individuals with Paget's Disease of the Bone to ensure adequate hydration, as this is fundamental to good health in general. Hydration is of utmost importance in sustaining numerous physiological processes, such as bone health, and can also aid in the management of certain symptoms linked to Paget's Disease.

An abnormal remodeling of bones characterizes Paget's Disease, resulting in bones that are weakened and deformed. Ensuring appropriate hydration is critical for preserving the structural integrity of bones and promoting the overall health of the musculoskeletal system. Bone tissue is predominantly composed of water, and progressive dehydration may contribute to a decline in bone density.

Moreover, joint health is significantly impacted by hydration, and those afflicted with Paget's Disease frequently endure joint discomfort and stiffness. Maintaining adequate hydration is beneficial for lubricating joints, which can facilitate movement and potentially alleviate pain associated with the condition.

The following are hydration guidelines for those afflicted with Paget's Disease:

1. Promote consistent hydration: Advocate for individuals to consume a sufficient quantity of water daily. Hydration is best achieved through the consumption of water, although the precise quantity required may differ depending on variables including age, weight, and level of physical activity.

2. Observe Hydration Levels: Observe for signs of dehydration, including parched mouth, vertigo,

and dark urine. These may suggest the need for additional fluids.

3. Consume Hydrating Foods: Certain fruits and vegetables are rich in water and can aid in hydration as a whole. Oranges, cucumber, and watermelon should be incorporated into the diet.

4. It is generally permissible to consume caffeinated and alcoholic beverages in moderation; however, excessive consumption of these substances can lead to dehydration. Promote the use of water in a balanced and moderate manner.

5. Tailored Hydration Strategies: Collaborate with healthcare practitioners to develop individualized hydration strategies that are by the unique requirements and medical background of each patient.

6. It is imperative to remind individuals with Paget's Disease to maintain adequate hydration before, during, and after physical activity. This is

of the utmost importance in maintaining bone health and averting dehydration.

7. Electrolyte balance is a factor that healthcare professionals may advise in certain situations, particularly when medications or conditions are implicated in the disturbance. In such cases, electrolyte-rich beverages may be suggested. However, this should be done under supervision so that sodium intake is not excessive.

Adequate hydration is a straightforward and efficacious method of promoting general well-being, particularly for Paget's Disease. Individuals should seek guidance from their healthcare team to ascertain the precise hydration requirements that are by their particular condition and general health condition.

CHAPTER FOUR

Planning Meals To Promote Bone Health In Patients With Paget's Disease

Due to the unique challenges that Paget's Disease of Bone presents to bone health, meal preparation is an essential component of managing the condition. A nutritious and balanced diet that is abundant in essential nutrients may aid in the preservation of bone density, alleviation of symptoms, and promotion of general health in people diagnosed with Paget's Disease.

The following elements are crucial to take into account when devising meal plans to promote optimal bone health:

1. Foods Rich in Calcium Calcium is an essential mineral for healthy bones. To ensure a sufficient calcium intake, incorporate dairy products, verdant green vegetables, tofu, and fortified plant-based milk into one's diet.

2. Sources of Vitamin D Vitamin D is a prerequisite for the absorption of calcium.

Incorporate vitamin D-rich foods into your diet, including fortified cereals, oily salmon, and egg yolks. Additionally, sunlight provides a natural source of vitamin D.

3. Protein is an indispensable nutrient for the maintenance of muscle health, thereby providing an indirect benefit to bone health. Consume lean sources of protein, such as poultry, fish, legumes, lean meats, and dairy products.

4. Vitamin K-Rich Foods: Bone metabolism is influenced by vitamin K. Broccoli, Brussels sprouts, and leafy green vegetables are all excellent sources of vitamin K.

5. Magnesium Inclusion: Due to its role in bone formation, magnesium may assist in the alleviation of Paget's Disease symptoms. Consume foods that are abundant in magnesium, including nuts, seeds, whole cereals, and leafy vegetables.

6. An inordinate consumption of phosphorus, which is vital for maintaining healthy bones, can

worsen the symptoms associated with Paget's Disease. Maintain a healthy balance of phosphorus-rich foods in your diet, such as legumes, dairy, and livestock.

7. Sufficient Fiber Consumption: A dietary regimen abundant in whole cereals, fruits, and vegetables supplies fiber, an essential nutrient that confers positive effects on overall health. Sufficient consumption of fiber promotes digestive health and potentially enhances the general well-being of people diagnosed with Paget's Disease.

8. Limit your intake of processed foods, as their high sodium content may contribute to bone loss. For the health of the bones, limiting the consumption of processed and salted foods can be beneficial.

9. Water retention: As previously stated, adequate hydration is vital for maintaining healthy bones.

Water contributes to the strength and density of bones by supporting their overall structure and function.

10.   Seeking   Advice   from   Healthcare Professionals: The nutritional requirements of individuals may differ depending on Paget's Disease severity and additional health-related variables.

Consistent   consultation   with   healthcare professionals, such as nutritionists or dietitians, guarantees that meal plans are customized to address particular requirements and objectives.

In summary, a meticulously devised meal regimen constitutes a beneficial element in the management of Paget's Disease of the Bone. Individuals can augment their general well-being and mitigate the consequences of Paget's Disease on their bones by prioritizing nutrient-dense foods that promote bone health and seeking guidance from healthcare experts.

Paget's Disease Of The Bone: A Fundamental Understanding

Paget's Disease of Bone is a persistent condition distinguished by atypical bone remodeling, which results in the enlargement and attenuation of bones. Distinguished by the initial description provided by Sir James Paget in 1877, this skeletal malady predominantly impacts the elderly population. It is hypothesized that genetic factors and viral infections contribute to its development, although the precise cause is still unknown.

Paget's Disease is characterized by an abnormal proliferation and degeneration of bone tissue. This causes bones to swell, deform, and become more susceptible to fractures. The long bones of the legs, spine, pelvis, and skull are frequently impacted bones. Complicated matters may manifest as discomfort spanning from mild to severe, deformities to neurological problems or hearing loss.

Frequently, a combination of clinical evaluations, imaging studies (e.g., X-rays), and blood tests measuring markers of bone turnover are utilized to diagnose Paget's Disease. Although no cure exists, the purpose of treatment is to prevent complications and alleviate symptoms. Commonly prescribed medications to reduce the risk of fractures and regulate bone turnover are bisphosphonates.

Adhering to Paget's Disease necessitates a holistic approach, encompassing adjustments to one's lifestyle, cooperation with healthcare practitioners, and resolution of frequently asked inquiries to augment comprehension and adaptive mechanisms.

Collaborative Efforts: Healthcare Professional Consultation

Effective management of Paget's Disease requires the active participation and cooperation of a multidisciplinary team of healthcare professionals, including patients. From the initial diagnosis to the ongoing management of the patient's condition, a multitude of specialists collaborate to develop an individualized care plan that is comprehensive in nature.

Rheumatologists contribute significantly to the understanding and management of Paget's Disease by their specialized knowledge in musculoskeletal disorders. Orthopedic surgeons may be consulted in instances where severe bone fractures or deformities occur. Pain management specialists provide assistance in the treatment of chronic pain that is a consequence of the ailment. Further, physical therapists develop exercise regimens to preserve range of motion and fortify the muscles that encircle the compromised bones.

Endocrinologists assist in the optimization of treatment strategies by monitoring the hormonal aspects of bone metabolism. Radiologists employ imaging modalities to detect alterations in the bone and evaluate the advancement of diseases. Consistent evaluations with primary care physicians are imperative for monitoring overall health and coordinating care.

Patients who engage in open communication and actively participate in healthcare decision-making are better equipped to navigate the intricate challenges associated with Paget's Disease. Collaborative endeavors transcend the realm of healthcare practitioners and encompass the assistance of family members, caregivers, and patient advocacy organizations. A unified approach guarantees a comprehensive and patient-centric experience in healthcare.

CHAPTER FIVE

Changes In Lifestyle Regarding Paget's Disease

Incorporating lifestyle adjustments is crucial for the effective management of Paget's Disease and the enhancement of one's overall quality of life. The purpose of these modifications is to mitigate symptoms, decrease the likelihood of complications, and improve both physical and emotional health.

Exercise and physical activity comprise 1. Walking and swimming are examples of low-impact activities that aid in the maintenance of bone strength and flexibility. Physical therapy may be advised to modify an exercise regimen to meet the specific requirements of the individual.

2. Nutrition: Sufficient consumption of calcium and vitamin D is critical for maintaining optimal bone health. Prescriptions for dietary supplements may be necessary to ensure adequate levels, particularly in cases of deficiency.

Health is promoted by a balanced diet that is abundant in fruits, vegetables, and lean proteins.

3. Fall Prevention: Fall prevention measures are of utmost importance as they mitigate the heightened risk of fractures. This includes exercising balance exercises, modifying the home environment to reduce stumbling hazards, and utilizing assistive devices.

4. Pain Management: paget's disease is frequently accompanied by chronic pain. Physical therapy, medications, and relaxation techniques are all viable options for the effective management of pain. Effective collaboration with healthcare providers is essential for customizing pain management strategies to meet the unique requirements of each patient.

5. Consistent Monitoring and Follow-up: Consistent consultations with healthcare practitioners are imperative for overseeing the advancement of the illness, evaluating the effectiveness of treatments, and attending to

emergent issues. Implementing this proactive approach enables the timely modification of the treatment plan.

Lifestyle adjustments enable individuals diagnosed with Paget's Disease to actively participate in their health, fostering resilience and improving their capacity to manage the difficulties presented by the condition.

FAQs: Frequently Asked Questions
Is Paget's Disease a hereditary condition?

A1: Although Paget's Disease does have a genetic component, it is not exclusively inherited. While specific genetic predispositions may exist, the condition can also be influenced by environmental factors and viral infections.

Can Paget's disease be remedied?

A2: At this time, a cure for Paget's Disease does not exist. Medication and lifestyle modifications are examples of effective management strategies that can be utilized to alleviate symptoms, avert complications, and enhance quality of life.

How is the diagnosis of Paget's Disease made?

A3: A comprehensive diagnostic approach generally incorporates clinical evaluations, imaging investigations (e.g., bone scans and X-rays), and blood analyses to quantify biomarkers of bone resorption.

For an accurate diagnosis, a comprehensive evaluation by a rheumatologist or other specialist is required.

Q4: Which drugs are prescribed for the treatment of Paget's Disease?

A4: Bisphosphonates are frequently prescribed to reduce the risk of fractures and regulate bone turnover. To manage symptoms, additional medications such as calcitonin or pain relievers may be prescribed. On the individual's overall health and the severity of the disease, treatment plans are customized.

Q5: Can modifications to one's lifestyle aid in the management of Paget's disease?

A5: Indeed, lifestyle modifications are of paramount importance in the management of Paget's Disease. Implementing a well-rounded regimen that includes a balanced diet, suitable exercise routine, fall prevention strategies, and consistent monitoring are all integral elements of an all-encompassing strategy for managing Paget's Disease.

Sixth, are support organizations available for those afflicted with Paget's disease?

A6: Indeed, patient advocacy organizations and support groups are specifically formed to address Paget's Disease.

Establishing connections with individuals who are confronted with comparable obstacles can yield invaluable perspectives, and emotional solace, and foster a sense of communal belonging. Frequently, healthcare practitioners can supply patients with details regarding nearby or digital support systems.

In summary, gaining a comprehensive understanding of Paget's Disease necessitates an exploration of its intricacies, a cooperative effort with healthcare practitioners, adjustments to one's lifestyle, and responses to frequently asked inquiries to equip individuals with the necessary information to effectively manage the condition.

Conclusion

Paget's Disease of Bone, an enduring condition distinguished by atypical bone tissue degeneration and regeneration, necessitates a comprehensive strategy for its management. The function of nutrition in promoting overall bone health among individuals who are affected is crucial. It is essential to maintain a well-balanced diet that is abundant in calcium and vitamin D, as these nutrients play a fundamental role in the process of bone remodeling and strength.

Fortified foods, dairy products, and leafy vegetables are all excellent sources of calcium. Vitamin D, on the other hand, can be obtained from fatty salmon, egg yolks, and sunlight exposure.

Furthermore, it can be advantageous to consume foods that are abundant in anti-inflammatory properties. Salmon and mackerel contain omega-3 fatty acids, which have demonstrated promise in the reduction of inflammation. By preventing oxidative stress, antioxidant-rich fruits and vegetables, including beets, spinach, and berries, also promote bone health.

Caffeine and foods high in sodium should be consumed in moderation, as they can inhibit the absorption of calcium and negatively impact bone health. It is recommended to maintain a moderate protein intake, as an excessive amount may contribute to calcium loss.

Additionally, incorporating bone-strengthening exercises under the supervision of a healthcare professional can be beneficial. Hydration is vital. It is of the utmost importance that people with Paget's Disease collaborate closely with healthcare professionals, such as dietitians, to customize dietary decisions that align with their unique health requirements and prescribed medications.

THE END